UNDERSTANDING CHRONIC MYELOID LEUKEMIA

DIAGNOSING IT, AND TREATING IT

DR. J.P JUDE

Table of Contents

CHAPTER ONE

INTRODUCTION

A kind of cancer that affects the bone marrow and blood is called chronic granulocytic leukemia (CGL), commonly referred to as chronic myeloid leukemia (CML). Granulocytes are a type of white blood cell that have an abnormally high quantity in CGL, especially in the early stages of the disease. The Philadelphia chromosome, a genetic anomaly caused by a reciprocal translocation of chromosomes 9 and 22, is the cause of this overproduction.

The Philadelphia chromosome, which results in the fusion gene BCR-ABL, is the defining characteristic of CGL. This fusion gene leads to the production of a protein with aberrant tyrosine kinase activity, which encourages unchecked cell division and proliferation. Fatigue, weakness, and an elevated risk of bleeding and infection can result from the unregulated expansion of white blood cells, which can push out normal blood cells in the bone marrow and reduce red blood cells and platelets.

Three phases are usually experienced by CGL progression: the chronic period, the accelerated phase, and the explosion phase. Patients may not have any symptoms at all or just have minor ones throughout the chronic period. The condition may progress to the accelerated phase, which is marked by a quicker rise in the white blood cell count and increased symptoms, if treatment is not received. The illness may eventually advance to the blast phase, where immature blast cells multiply quickly and resemble acute leukemia.

The available CGL treatments have changed dramatically in recent years. For many individuals with chronic-phase CGL, targeted treatments such tyrosine kinase inhibitors (TKIs) are a successful first-line treatment that effectively controls the disease. Patients in advanced stages of the disease or those who are not responsive to or cannot take TKIs may benefit from stem cell transplantation.

Assessing therapy response and disease progression requires routine blood count monitoring and molecular testing for BCR-ABL levels. Many CGL patients can now experience long-term remission and have happy lives with appropriate medical management thanks to breakthroughs in treatment.

The pathophysiological understanding

The Philadelphia chromosome is a genetic anomaly that is central to the pathogenesis of Chronic Granulocytic Leukemia (CGL), often referred to as Chronic Myeloid Leukemia (CML). The Abelson (ABL) gene on chromosome 9 and the breakpoint cluster region (BCR) gene on chromosome 22 fuse as a result of a reciprocal translocation between chromosomes 9 and 22, resulting in this chromosomal anomaly.

A constitutively active tyrosine kinase protein is produced by the hybrid gene known as BCR-ABL, which is created when the ABL and BCR genes fuse. Because it promotes unchecked cell proliferation, inhibits apoptosis (programmed cell death), and interferes with normal cellular signaling pathways, this aberrant protein is crucial to the pathophysiology of CGL.

The phosphoinositide 3-kinase (PI3K)/Akt pathway and the Ras/mitogen-activated protein kinase (MAPK) pathway are two downstream signaling pathways that are triggered by the BCR-ABL protein. These pathways control various biological functions, including migration, survival, differentiation, and cell proliferation. Excessive production and accumulation of immature myeloid cells, especially granulocytes, in the bone marrow and peripheral circulation are caused by dysregulation of these pathways.

A number of clinical symptoms, including as leukocytosis (an increased white blood cell count), splenomegaly (enlargement of the spleen), and anemia (low red blood cell count) are caused by the overproduction of granulocytes in CGL. Furthermore, a higher concentration of immature white blood cells compromises immunological function and puts patients at risk for infections.

Three phases are usually experienced by CGL progression: the chronic period, the accelerated phase, and the explosion phase. The disease's moderate symptoms and comparatively steady blood levels are hallmarks of the chronic phase. On the other hand, CGL can enter the accelerated phase, which is marked by a faster pace of disease progression, more blast cell proliferation, and deteriorating symptoms, if it is not treated or is not managed well. In the end, the illness could progress to the blast phase, which would resemble acute leukemia and be characterized by a high concentration of immature blast cells in the peripheral blood and bone marrow.

The development of targeted medicines, including tyrosine kinase inhibitors (TKIs), which directly target the BCR-ABL protein and have transformed the treatment of this disease, has been made possible thanks to better understanding of the underlying pathophysiology of CGL. TKIs successfully regulate the proliferation of leukemic cells and produce remission in a significant number of CGL patients by blocking BCR-ABL activity.

Presentation of Clinical Data

Depending on the patient's unique traits and the disease's stage, Chronic Granulocytic Leukemia (CGL), also known as Chronic Myeloid Leukemia (CML), might manifest differently clinically. An outline of the typical clinical signs and symptoms connected to each stage of CGL is provided below:

Chronic Stage:

frequently asymptomatic and may only be discovered by chance when doing regular blood work.

When symptoms do occur, they are typically vague and mild, and they include weakness, weariness, and pain in the abdomen (from splenomegaly).

Splenomegaly, or splenic enlargement, is a common occurrence that can lead to discomfort in the left upper quadrant, early satiety, and stomach fullness.

A low-grade temperature, nocturnal sweats, and inadvertent weight loss are possible side effects for certain patients.

Phase Accelerated:

represents a stage of the disease that progresses and whose symptoms get worse, lying between the chronic and blast stages.

In the chronic phase, patients may notice a rise in the frequency and intensity of their symptoms.

It's possible for leukocytosis—an elevated white blood cell count—to go worse and for blast cells to start showing up in the bone marrow and peripheral circulation.

Anemia (low red blood cell count) and thrombocytopenia (low platelet count) may worsen, increasing the risk of bleeding and exhaustion.

Phase of Blast:

symbolizes a change into a state resembling acute leukemia, with a high concentration of blast cells in the peripheral blood and bone marrow.

Acute leukemia symptoms that patients may experience include fever, bone pain, bleeding, easy bruising, and indications of organ infiltration, such as lymphadenopathy, hepatomegaly, and splenomegaly.

Fast-moving sickness and a decline in general health are hallmarks of the blast phase.

Individuals diagnosed with blast phase CGL need to start receiving intensive treatment very away, which may include stem cell transplantation, targeted therapy, or chemotherapy.

Laboratory studies are essential for both identifying and tracking CGL in addition to clinical manifestations. Typically, peripheral blood tests show possible anemia, thrombocytosis (high platelet count), and leukocytosis with a left shift (increased immature white blood cells). To confirm the diagnosis and determine the stage of the disease, a bone marrow aspiration and biopsy are required.

Making informed treatment decisions and enhancing patient outcomes need early detection and precise staging of CGL. Many CGL patients can now achieve long-term remission and lead happy lives with appropriate medical care thanks to developments in targeted therapy. To evaluate the effectiveness of treatment and the course of the disease, regular monitoring of blood counts and symptoms is crucial.

Diagnostic Assessment

In order to diagnose Chronic Granulocytic Leukemia (CGL), commonly referred to as Chronic Myeloid Leukemia (CML), a combination of molecular research, laboratory testing, and clinical examination is used. This is a synopsis of the diagnostic methodology:

Clinical Evaluation:

A comprehensive medical history and physical examination are frequently the first steps in the diagnosis process.

Signs of bleeding or infection, weakness, exhaustion, splenomegaly-related stomach discomfort, and accidental weight loss are among the clinical symptoms suggestive of CGL.

Evaluation of the liver, spleen, and lymph nodes is crucial since hepatomegaly and splenomegaly are frequent observations in CGL.

Laboratory Examinations:

A complete blood count (CBC) with differential usually reveals a left shift (more immature granulocytes) and leukocytosis (an increased white blood cell count).

CHAPTER TWO

There may also be anemia (low red blood cell count) and thrombocytosis (high platelet count).

Examining a peripheral blood smear can reveal a higher concentration of immature myeloid cells, such as promyelocytes, myeloblasts, and myelocytes.

Aspiration and biopsy of the bone marrow: Crucial for verifying the diagnosis and determining the proportion of blasts, cellularity, and Philadelphia chromosome presence. Determining the disease phase (chronic, accelerated, or blast phase) is another benefit of bone marrow investigation.

Molecular studies: The identification of the BCR-ABL fusion gene and/or Philadelphia chromosome is essential for the diagnosis of CGL. Common molecular approaches for determining the location of the Philadelphia chromosome and measuring BCR-ABL transcripts are polymerase chain reaction (PCR) and fluorescence in situ hybridization (FISH), respectively.

Imaging Research:

A computed tomography (CT) scan or abdominal ultrasound is helpful in determining the size of the liver and spleen, identifying hepatomegaly and splenomegaly, and testing for lymphadenopathy.

Skeletal survey: X-rays of the bones might be taken to check for lytic lesions or bone discomfort, which can appear in later stages of the illness.

Extra Examinations:

Using flow cytometry, leukemic cells can be immunophenotyped to determine their myeloid lineage and check for abnormal antigen expression.

Cytogenetic analysis: This method can identify additional chromosomal abnormalities that may have prognostic significance in addition to detecting the Philadelphia chromosome.

Quantitative PCR for BCR-ABL monitoring: Following diagnosis, tracking BCR-ABL transcript levels on a frequent basis is essential for determining how well a treatment is working and how far along the disease is.

To accurately diagnose CGL, determine the disease's stage, and inform treatment choices, a thorough diagnostic assessment is necessary. For the best care of patients with CGL, cooperation between hematologists, oncologists, pathologists, and other medical professionals is essential.

Prognostic factors and risk stratification

Identifying prognostic variables and risk stratification are essential in directing therapy choices and forecasting results for Chronic Granulocytic Leukemia (CGL), sometimes referred to as Chronic Myeloid Leukemia

(CML). The following are some crucial elements of risk prognostication and stratification:

Stage of Illness:

One important predictor of prognosis is the stage of the disease at diagnosis. When compared to patients diagnosed in the rapid or blast phase, those diagnosed in the chronic phase typically experience better outcomes.

Molecular and Cytogenetic Abnormalities:

The prognosis may be affected by the presence of additional chromosomal abnormalities in addition to the Philadelphia chromosome. Poorer outcomes are linked to specific chromosomal abnormalities, including trisomy 8, deletions in the long arm of chromosome 7, and complicated karyotypes.

Important prognostic information can be obtained by quantifying BCR-ABL transcript levels using molecular methods like quantitative PCR. Increased BCR-ABL transcript levels at diagnosis or throughout treatment could be a sign of a worse response to therapy and a more aggressive course of the disease.

Reaction to Medication:

Long-term results are strongly predicted by early response to treatment, as measured by reduction in BCR-ABL transcript levels (e.g., molecular response milestones). Securing profound and long-lasting chemical reactions is linked to enhanced overall and progression-free survival.

Poorer results are linked to resistance to tyrosine kinase inhibitors (TKIs), which is manifested by inability to reach or sustain molecular response benchmarks. Making decisions about treatment and prognosis is also influenced by the discovery of TKI-resistant mutations in the BCR-ABL kinase domain.

Age and Level of Performance:

Poorer performance status at diagnosis and older age are typically linked to worse outcomes. Patients who are elderly or have substantial comorbidities may not be able to tolerate intense therapy as well as face more side effects from treatment.

Symptom Burden and Spleen Size:

The degree and existence of splenomegaly at diagnosis may indicate the severity of the illness and have an impact on prognosis. Bad results are linked to larger spleen sizes (>10 cm below the costal border).

Fatigue, weight loss, and constitutional symptoms are examples of symptom burden that can affect prognosis and quality of life.

Complications and Comorbidities:

Comorbid conditions like diabetes, cardiovascular disease, and renal impairment might affect a patient's prognosis and options for therapy.

Treatment results and overall survival may be impacted by the emergence of treatment-related problems include myelosuppression, infections, and vascular events.

Reaction to Treatment and Illness Monitoring:

Prognosis and treatment decision-making depend on routinely evaluating response to therapy using serial peripheral blood count tests, bone marrow examination, and molecular monitoring of BCR-ABL transcript levels.

Healthcare practitioners can enhance patient outcomes for CGL patients by customizing treatment regimens and surveillance protocols based on these risk factors and prognostic markers. Hematologists, oncologists, molecular biologists, and other medical specialists must work closely together to provide patients with CGL with tailored therapy and monitoring.

Methods of Therapy

With the development of targeted medicines during the past few decades, the management of Chronic Granulocytic Leukemia (CGL), also known as Chronic Myeloid Leukemia (CML), has undergone significant change. The following are the primary methods of treating CGL:

TKIs, or tyrosine kinase inhibitors:

The mainstay of CGL treatment is a combination of TKIs and targeted targeting of the BCR-ABL tyrosine kinase protein, which promotes leukemic cell growth.

Imatinib is one of the first-generation TKIs; it was the first to be authorized for the treatment of CML. Dasatinib, nilotinib, and bosutinib are examples of second-generation TKIs that have increased potency and effectiveness against BCR-ABL, especially against specific mutations linked to TKI resistance.

The T315I mutation, which causes resistance to older TKIs, is one of the many BCR-ABL mutations that third-generation TKIs, like ponatinib, are successful against.

For individuals with a diagnosis of CGL in the chronic phase, TKIs are usually the first line of treatment. Additionally, they work well to slow down the course of the illness and put patients with rapid or blast phase CGL into remission.

Stem Cell Replacement Therapy:

Certain CGL patients may be candidates for allogeneic hematopoietic stem cell transplantation (HSCT), especially if they have severe illness or have not responded well to TKIs.

By substituting healthy donor stem cells for the damaged bone marrow, HSCT provides the possibility of long-term disease control or cure. Nevertheless, there are considerable hazards involved, such as graft-versus-host disease and transplant-related complications (GVHD).

Assistive Healthcare:

Supportive care practices are essential for controlling the side effects and symptoms of CGL and its treatment.

Red blood cell transfusions for anemia patients, platelet transfusions for thrombocytopenia patients, and antibiotic prophylaxis to prevent infections are examples of supportive treatment.

Growth factors that increase the formation of white blood cells and lower the risk of infection include granulocyte colony-stimulating factor (G-CSF).

Clinical Examinations:

Patients who meet the eligibility requirements may choose to take part in clinical trials, especially those who have refractory disease or are interested in trying out new treatment modalities.

To enhance treatment outcomes and minimize side effects, clinical studies may explore novel TKIs, combination treatments, immunotherapies, or other targeted medicines.

Observation and observation:

It is imperative to conduct routine monitoring of treatment response and disease progression in order to optimize patient outcomes for CGL patients.

Peripheral blood count assessments, bone marrow evaluations, and molecular monitoring of BCR-ABL transcript levels using methods like quantitative PCR are some examples of monitoring methods.

A patient's age, comorbidities, cytogenetic and molecular risk factors, responsiveness to treatment, and disease stage are all taken into consideration while determining a course of treatment for CGL. Hematologists, oncologists, transplant experts, and other medical professionals must work closely together to create individualized treatment programs and offer complete care for patients with CGL.

An essential part of treating Chronic Granulocytic Leukemia (CGL), sometimes referred to as Chronic Myeloid Leukemia (CML), is monitoring and response evaluation. In order to detect illness development, evaluate treatment efficacy, and inform therapeutic decisions, regular monitoring is helpful. An outline of the essential elements of CGL's reaction evaluation and monitoring is provided below:

Circumstantial Blood Counts:

It is imperative to conduct routine complete blood count (CBC) monitoring with differential to evaluate alterations in leukocyte, erythrocyte, and platelet counts.

CBC monitoring is useful in assessing medication response, identifying treatment-related toxicities, and detecting cytopenias, such as anemia, thrombocytopenia, and neutropenia, in patients undergoing treatment.

Assessment of Bone Marrow:

As part of the diagnostic process and to monitor the disease's progression and response to treatment, bone marrow aspiration and biopsy may be done on a regular basis.

CHAPTER THREE

Bone marrow samples can be morphologically assessed to ascertain the percentage of blasts, level of cell differentiation, and existence of treatment-related alterations.

Monitoring BCR-ABL Transcript Levels Molecularly:

BCR-ABL transcript levels in peripheral blood samples are determined using the quantitative polymerase chain reaction (PCR) or other molecular methods.

At the molecular level, molecular monitoring enables accurate assessment of therapy response and quantification of residual disease burden.

Molecular response milestones, which are used to assess the effectiveness of treatment, are determined based on predefined thresholds for BCR-ABL transcript levels. Examples of these milestones are major molecular response (MMR) and deep molecular response (DMR).

Analysis of Cytogenesis:

The Philadelphia chromosome and other cytogenetic alterations can be found in bone marrow cells by cytogenetic analysis.

An essential part of evaluating response in CGL is cytogenetic response, which is measured by calculating the proportion of Philadelphia chromosome-positive metaphases in bone marrow samples.

Imaging Research:

For the purpose of tracking alterations in the size of the spleen and identifying extramedullary disease involvement (such as hepatomegaly or lymphadenopathy), abdominal ultrasonography or computed tomography (CT) scans may be utilized.

Particularly in individuals with advanced disease, skeletal imaging (such as X-rays, magnetic resonance imaging [MRI], and bone scans) may be carried out to assess for bone involvement or lytic lesions.

Clinical Evaluation and Symptom Observation:

Monitoring symptoms associated with the disease, side effects of treatment, and general patient well-being all depend on routine clinical assessment.

Patient-reported outcomes, such as symptom scores and quality of life evaluations, can offer important information about the burden of the condition and how tolerable the treatment is.

Reaction Standards:

Standardized criteria, such as those developed by the National Comprehensive Cancer Network (NCCN) or European LeukemiaNet (ELN), provide the basis for response assessment in CGL.

Response criteria are used to guide treatment decisions and put patients into different response categories (e.g., optimal response, warning, failure) based on molecular, cytogenetic, and hematological characteristics.

Optimizing outcomes for CGL patients requires thorough and frequent monitoring of the illness state and response to treatment. Hematologists, oncologists, laboratory specialists, and other healthcare professionals must work closely together to evaluate monitoring data, modify treatment plans, and give patients with CGL individualized care.

Handling Adverse Events Associated with Treatment

When patients with Chronic Granulocytic Leukemia (CGL) are receiving therapy, especially with tyrosine kinase inhibitors (TKIs) or other therapeutic modalities, managing treatment-related adverse events (AEs) is an essential element of their care. The following list of typical treatment-related side effects includes management techniques for each:

Myelosuppression

One of the most frequent side effects of TKIs is myelosuppression, which includes thrombocytopenia, anemia, and neutropenia.

To provide for the recovery of blood counts, management may entail changing the TKI's dosage or stopping it altogether.

When necessary, supportive care interventions can be used, such as platelet transfusions for thrombocytopenia, red blood cell transfusions for anemia, and hematopoietic growth factors (such as granulocyte colony-stimulating factor [G-CSF] for neutropenia).

Intestinal Toxicology:

TKIs may cause gastrointestinal adverse effects as nausea, vomiting, diarrhea, and abdominal pain.

Antiemetic drugs for nausea and vomiting, antidiarrheal pharmaceuticals for diarrhea, and proton pump inhibitors or H2-receptor antagonists for the control of stomach acid are examples of symptomatic therapy.

TKI side effects may be lessened by encouraging patients to take them with meals or a full glass of water.

Rash on the Skin:

One of the most frequent side effects of certain TKIs, like dasatinib and nilotinib, is skin rash.

For mild to moderate rash, topical corticosteroids and emollients may offer symptomatic relief.

In extreme situations, it could be required to lower the dosage or temporarily stop taking the offending TKI, and then re-escalate it when the rash goes away.

Retention of Fluid and Peripheral Edema:

Certain TKIs, such dasatinib, might result in peripheral edema and fluid retention.

Diuretics can be used to treat patients' fluid retention if they experience severe peripheral edema or respiratory problems.

In severe cases, or if supportive measures are not enough to control the symptoms, the TKI may need to be stopped altogether or its dose reduced.

Cardiovascular Hazard:

TKIs have been linked to cardiovascular toxicities such as hypertension, QT prolongation, and arterial thrombotic events, especially nilotinib and ponatinib.

For patients on TKIs, blood pressure monitoring and antihypertensive drug management of hypertension are crucial.

To treat QT prolongation, electrocardiogram (ECG) monitoring and electrolyte imbalance correction may be required.

Patients at high risk of arterial thrombotic events may be evaluated for antiplatelet treatment and thromboprophylaxis.

Hepatotoxicity:

Certain TKIs, such ponatinib, can cause hepatotoxicity and elevated liver enzymes.

If liver enzyme elevations are substantial or chronic, dose modifications or stopping the TKI may be necessary. Liver function tests should be performed on a regular basis.

Additional Unfavorable Events

Additional side effects linked to TKIs include headaches, weariness, musculoskeletal pain, and irregular electrolytes.

These symptoms may be best managed symptomatically with analgesics, rest, and fluids.

Optimizing treatment results and quality of life in CGL patients requires aggressive management of symptoms and close observation of patients for treatment-related side events. Throughout the duration of treatment, healthcare professionals should inform patients about possible side effects, promote candid discussion about symptoms, and offer supportive care measures as needed.

Long-Term Supervision and Survival

For patients with Chronic Granulocytic Leukemia (CGL), sometimes called Chronic Myeloid Leukemia (CML), who have reached remission or stable disease control, long-term treatment and survivorship care are crucial. The following are important facets of survivorship treatment and long-term management:

Frequent Visits for Follow-Up:

Patients should see their doctors for follow-up appointments on a regular basis; at first, this should be every three to six months, but as the disease stabilizes, this frequency should decrease.

Follow-up appointments enable tracking the state of the condition, evaluating the effectiveness of the treatment, identifying any progression or recurrence of the illness, and managing any side effects or late effects of the treatment.

Molecular Surveillance:

Quantitative PCR-based molecular monitoring of BCR-ABL transcript levels in peripheral blood is crucial for determining therapy response, identifying molecular relapse, and informing treatment choices.

Although the level of surveillance may be lowered for patients who achieve deep molecular responses (such as undetectable BCR-ABL transcripts), they should nonetheless go for routine follow-up appointments to keep an eye out for any possible disease return.

Hematologic and Cytogenetic Evaluations:

To check for cytogenetic reactions and gauge bone marrow remission, periodic bone marrow evaluations and cytogenetic analyses may be carried out.

Regular monitoring of complete blood counts (CBC) with differential is necessary to identify variations in blood cell counts and evaluate potential indicators of illness progression or treatment-related problems.

Sustaining TKI Therapy:

For the purpose of preventing disease relapse and maintaining remission, patients who receive and maintain excellent responses to TKI therapy should continue treatment permanently.

To optimize treatment success, patients should be informed about the significance of taking their medication as directed. Adherence to TKI therapy is essential.

Handling Therapy-Related Late Effects:

Chronic TKI treatment may result in cumulative toxicities and late consequences, such as musculoskeletal issues, metabolic irregularities, cardiovascular problems, and secondary cancers.

Patients should be kept an eye out for late-effect indicators and symptoms, and suitable measures should be taken to control and lessen these issues.

Promoting Health and Preventing Diseases:

Promoting healthy lifestyle practices is crucial for enhancing general health and wellbeing. These practices include frequent exercise, a balanced diet, quitting smoking, and moderate alcohol consumption.

To lower the risk of subsequent cancers and infectious problems, patients should be informed about the significance of cancer screening and vaccine recommendations.

Programs for Survivorship and Psychosocial Support:

Patients might benefit from psychosocial support services, like support groups, counseling, and survivorship programs, to help them deal with the practical, social, and emotional difficulties of living with and beyond cancer.

Survivorship care plans can help with coordinated care and communication amongst healthcare professionals by providing information about the patient's treatment history, follow-up schedule, potential late effects, and suggestions for ongoing care.

A multidisciplinary strategy comprising hematologists, oncologists, primary care physicians, nurses, social workers, and other healthcare professionals is necessary for the long-term management and survivorship care of patients with CGL. Healthcare professionals can improve the long-term results and quality of life for patients with CGL by attending to the physical, emotional, and practical requirements of survivors.

Treatment Termination and Remission Without Therapy

In the management of Chronic Granulocytic Leukemia (CGL), also known as Chronic Myeloid Leukemia (CML), stopping treatment and reaching therapy-free remission have become crucial objectives. This is especially true for patients who have demonstrated long-lasting and profound molecular responses to tyrosine kinase inhibitor (TKI) therapy. An outline of therapy cessation and therapy-free remission in CGL is shown below:

Choice of Patient:

Patients who have achieved and maintained deep molecular responses—defined as a persistent decline in BCR-ABL transcript levels below a predefined threshold (e.g., MR4.5 or deeper) for a specific duration—are often candidates for therapy-free remission and the cessation of treatment.

The absence of substantial comorbidities, stable blood counts, the absence of disease progression, and the patient's willingness to receive close monitoring are possible additional variables to take into account.

Trials of Discontinuation:

Discontinuation trials have shown that it is feasible and safe to stop TKI therapy in a subset of patients who have achieved deep molecular responses. Examples of these trials are STIM (Stop Imatinib) and TWISTER (Tasigna or nilotinib Withdrawal in Stable Chronic Myeloid Leukemia Patients in Molecular Response).

Results from these trials have demonstrated that a portion of patients can sustain treatment-free remission (TFR) without the illness worsening or reoccurring for extended periods of time.

Observing During TFR:

When TKI therapy is stopped, patients are closely watched for any indications of a clinical relapse or molecular recurrence.

Quantitative PCR is used to monitor BCR-ABL transcript levels in peripheral blood at regular intervals (e.g., monthly for the first year, then every three months after that) in order to look for signs of molecular relapse.

Periodic clinical assessments, such as complete blood counts, physical exams, and symptom evaluations, should also be performed on patients.

Controlling Molecular Relapse:

Molecular relapse, which is characterized by the return of detectable BCR-ABL transcripts over a certain threshold, can happen to certain patients after treatment is stopped.

CHAPTER FOUR

For patients who experience a molecular relapse, it is advised to promptly resume TKI medication as early intervention can help restore molecular responses and stop the disease from progressing.

Factors Affecting TFR's Success:

Achieving deeper molecular responses (MR4.5 or deeper) before stopping treatment, maintaining the molecular response for a longer period of time, not having any further chromosomal abnormalities, and having low-risk Sokal or EUTOS scores are all factors linked to successful TFR.

Successful TFR outcomes also depend on close monitoring protocol adherence, patient compliance with follow-up visits and molecular testing, and continued patient education and support.

Current Research and Upcoming Paths:

The best practices for TFR and therapy termination in CGL are still being researched.

Novel strategies, including immune-based medicines, combination therapy, and treatment duration optimization, are being investigated in clinical trials to increase the possibility of attaining and sustaining TFR while lowering the risk of disease recurrence.

In the management of CGL, stopping treatment and reaching TFR are important turning points that, for some patients, may result in longer stretches of disease control without medication and better quality of life. In this rapidly changing profession, improving our understanding and maximizing results depends on continuous research, strict adherence to monitoring methods, and close collaboration between healthcare practitioners and patients.

Salvage and Relapse Treatments

Relapse in treatment-free remission (TFR) or chronic granulocytic leukemia (CGL), often called chronic myeloid leukemia (CML), happens when the disease reappears after a period of remission, usually after stopping tyrosine kinase inhibitor (TKI) therapy. Relapsed or resistant diseases can be managed using salvage therapy. An outline of salvage and relapse treatments for CGL is provided below:

The meaning of relapse

When CGL patients achieve treatment-free remission (TFR) or deep molecular response (DMR), relapse is generally defined as the return of detectable BCR-ABL transcripts over a predetermined threshold (e.g., $\geq 0.1\%$ on the International Scale).

Relapse can happen as a result of stopping treatment, having a poor reaction to TKI therapy, or developing TKI resistance because BCR-ABL mutations have emerged.

Handling Relapse:

In order to stop the progression of the disease and retain the best possible treatment results, relapse must be promptly detected and managed.

Prior to starting salvage therapy, recurrence must be confirmed by molecular monitoring of BCR-ABL transcript levels in bone marrow or peripheral blood.

Options for salvage therapy vary depending on the stage of the disease, previous treatment history, TKI resistance profile, patient comorbidities, and personal preferences of the patient.

Options for Salvage Therapy:

Changing to a Different TKI: Changing to a different TKI with an alternate mode of action or activity against particular BCR-ABL mutations may be beneficial in situations of relapse or TKI resistance. Salvation treatments often involve the use of TKIs from the second or third generation (e.g., ponatinib, dasatinib, nilotinib).

TKI Combinations: To overcome resistance and increase treatment efficacy, combining TKIs with distinct modes of action or adding additional medicines, like interferon-alpha, may be considered salvage therapy.

Allogeneic stem cell transplantation, or allo-SCT: This salvage therapy may be an option for patients with refractory or advanced illness, especially those with blast phase CGL or TKI-resistant mutations.

Investigational Therapies: Patients with relapsed or refractory CGL may benefit from new salvage therapy options by taking part in research studies examining innovative targeted medicines, immunotherapies, or combination regimens.

Supportive Care: In order to enhance patients' quality of life and general wellbeing, salvage therapy must incorporate supportive care measures, such as symptom management, treatment-related problems, and psychosocial support.

Tracking Salvage Therapy Reaction:

To determine the effectiveness of treatment, track the development of the disease, and modify treatment plans as appropriate, salvage therapy response must be regularly monitored.

To monitor the state of the disease and the response to treatment, cytogenetic analyses, clinical assessments, and molecular monitoring of BCR-ABL transcript levels are carried out on a regular basis.

Multidisciplinary Method:

A multidisciplinary strategy comprising hematologists, oncologists, transplant specialists, molecular biologists, and supportive care providers is necessary for the management of relapsed or refractory CGL.

Optimizing salvage therapy outcomes requires individualized treatment plans that are based on the unique characteristics of each patient's condition, past medical history, and desired level of care.

Relapse in CGL is a serious problem, but many patients can achieve sustained responses and keep the disease under control because to the availability of multiple salvage therapy choices and ongoing research efforts. Improved long-term results and successful management of recurrent or refractory disease require close collaboration between patients and healthcare professionals.

Summary

In conclusion, Philadelphia chromosome and BCR-ABL fusion gene presence are hallmarks of Chronic Granulocytic Leukemia (CGL), sometimes called Chronic Myeloid Leukemia (CML), a hematologic malignancy. The therapy of CGL has been revolutionized by the introduction of targeted medicines, specifically tyrosine kinase inhibitors (TKIs), as a result of advances in understanding the molecular etiology of the illness.

With the advent of TKIs, CGL patients are now able to achieve deep molecular responses and even drug-free remission, greatly improving treatment outcomes and overall survival. But issues including illness recurrence, resistance to treatment, and handling treatment-related side effects continue to be crucial factors in the long-term care of CGL patients.

Accurate diagnosis, risk assessment, choice of suitable treatment plans, tracking of treatment response, and proactive handling of treatment-related problems are essential components in managing CGL. Long-term survivorship care, which includes techniques for treatment termination, therapy-free remission, and management of recurrent or refractory disease, is also included in efforts to optimize patient outcomes.

To provide patients with CGL with comprehensive and personalized care, a multidisciplinary approach including hematologists, oncologists, transplant specialists, molecular biologists, and supportive care providers is necessary. Research into CGL biology is still being done in order to better understand the disease, find new targets for treatment, and help patients with this difficult condition.

Patients with CGL have a greater chance of long-term illness control and improved quality of life thanks to ongoing developments in treatment modalities, tailored medicine strategies, and supportive care interventions.

THE END